FOURTH EDITION

FACILITATOR'S GUIDE

Johns Hopkins
Evidence-Based Practice for Nurses and Healthcare Professionals

Model and Guidelines

Textbook available from SigmaMarketplace.org/Books and other book retailers

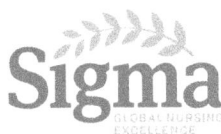

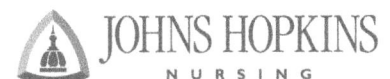

Sigma
GLOBAL NURSING EXCELLENCE

JOHNS HOPKINS
NURSING

Sigma Theta Tau International Honor Society of Nursing (Sigma) is a nonprofit organization whose mission is developing nurse leaders anywhere to improve healthcare everywhere. Founded in 1922, Sigma has more than 135,000 active members in over 100 countries and territories. Members include practicing nurses, instructors, researchers, policymakers, entrepreneurs, and others. Sigma's more than 540 chapters are located at more than 700 institutions of higher education throughout Armenia, Australia, Botswana, Brazil, Canada, Colombia, Croatia, England, Eswatini, Ghana, Hong Kong, Ireland, Israel, Italy, Jamaica, Japan, Jordan, Kenya, Lebanon, Malawi, Mexico, the Netherlands, Nigeria, Pakistan, Philippines, Portugal, Puerto Rico, Scotland, Singapore, South Africa, South Korea, Sweden, Taiwan, Tanzania, Thailand, the United States, and Wales. Learn more at www. sigmanursing.org.

Sigma Theta Tau International
550 West North Street
Indianapolis, IN, USA 46202

ISBN: 9781646480593
EPUB ISBN: 9781646480548

To request a review copy for course adoption, order additional books, buy in bulk, or purchase for corporate use, contact Sigma Marketplace at 888.654.4968 (US/Canada toll-free), +1.317.687.2256 (International), or solutions@ sigmamarketplace.org.

To request author information, or for speaker or other media requests, contact Sigma Marketing at 888.634.7575 (US/Canada toll-free) or +1.317.634.8171 (International).

FOURTH EDITION

FACILITATOR'S GUIDE

Johns Hopkins
Evidence-Based Practice for Nurses and Healthcare Professionals

Model and Guidelines

Judith Ascenzi, DNP, RN, CCRN-K
Kim Bissett, PhD, MBA, RN
Deborah Busch, DNP, MSN, RN, CPNP-PC, IBCLC
Sandra Dearholt, DNP, RN, NEA-BC
Madeleine Whalen, MSN/MPH, RN, CEN

Special acknowledgment to past contributors: Hayley D. Mark, PhD, MPH, RN, FAAN; Hyunjeong Park, PhD, MPH, MSN, RN; Sharon Dudley-Brown, PhD, APRN, BC, FNP; Mary Terhaar, DNSc, RN, CNS

Table of Contents

Part 1 Introduction to the Facilitator's Guide 5

Part 2 Baccalaureate Education 7

Part 3 Master's Education 11
Application of Research to Practice Course 11
Integration of EBP Into Master's Clinical Courses 13
Master's-Level Scholarly Project 13

Part 4 Doctoral Education 15
A Primer on EBP 16
Using the PICO in Education 16
Searching, Reviewing, and Appraising the Literature 16
Organizing and Presenting the Evidence 17
Teaching Models and Metrics 17

Part 5 Professional Development for Healthcare
Organizations 25
Instilling the Basics 25
Building EBP Capacity 25
Learning Needs Assessment 26
Identification of Teaching Methods 26
Fanning the Flame 30
Journal Clubs 30
Preceptor as EBP Mentor 31
Core EBP Continuing Education 31
Facilitated Protocol Development 32
Conclusion 32

Appendix Sample DNP Scholarly Project Curriculum Outline: Evidence-
Based Practice (EBP) Practice Question-Evidence-Translation
(PET) Pathway and Competencies for DNP Scholarly Projects . . . 37
Project Course #1: Practice Question/Problem Statement and Stakeholder
Identification 39
Project Course #2: Exploring the Evidence 41
Project Course #3: Connecting the Evidence for Project Translation 42
Project Course #4: Translation of Project Action Plan 45
Project Course #5: Evaluation of the Translation and Dissemination: 47

Reference Materials 49

Part 1
Introduction to the
Facilitator's Guide

Johns Hopkins Evidence-Based Practice for Nurses and Healthcare Professionals: Model and Guidelines, Fourth Edition, reaffirms the original mission of the Johns Hopkins Evidence-Based Practice (JHEBP) Model to support patient safety, professional development, and the education of healthcare students. Many evidence-based practice (EBP) books are in print today, but what makes this book valuable is its applicability for use in the classroom and its practical approach for the practice setting. The detailed guidelines and specific tools that accompany each step in the process promote success.

This Facilitator's Guide is intended for use by university faculty and nurses and healthcare clinicians facilitating professional development in healthcare organizations. *Johns Hopkins Evidence-Based Practice for Nurses and Healthcare Professionals: Model and Guidelines,* Fourth Edition, is used as a text for undergraduate, graduate, and doctoral courses to help students achieve the knowledge, skills, and abilities necessary to learn the essentials of their educational programs. The JHEBP Model is also used in the practice environment to guide clinical inquiry and enhance practice decision-making. The model and tools have high utility in both environments.

Parts 2, 3, and 4 of this guide offer details about incorporating EBP content throughout baccalaureate, master's, and doctoral curricula. They include suggestions about teaching EBP, leveling the content depending on student knowledge and previous experience with EBP, and examples of course objectives, assignments, and grading rubrics. Part 5 provides a discussion and practical examples for infusing EBP throughout an organization. We hope that you will find this guide a useful and exciting addition to the book.

Part 2
Baccalaureate Education

Evidence-based practice (EBP) is one of the American Association of Colleges of Nursing's *Essentials of Baccalaureate Education for Professional Nursing Practice* because professional nursing practice is grounded in the translation of current evidence into one's practice (www. aacnnursing.org/Portals/42/Publications/BaccEssentials08.pdf). EBP, an organizing structure to examine nursing practice, should be integrated into all aspects of undergraduate nursing education. In undergraduate-level nursing programs, EBP is often introduced in the first-semester course about the role of a professional nurse. It may then be threaded throughout the curriculum in didactic and clinical courses. EBP and research skills, including research methodology, the EBP process, and its application to a clinical question, may be taught in the second semester. As students expand their clinical skills in the third semester, they may continue to examine evidence for nursing practice at their clinical sites. In some programs in the fourth semester, students are required to take a seminar course that involves completion of an EBP project.

Nursing students often find it difficult to understand the concept of EBP and are challenged to apply it in a meaningful way because of their inexperience in practice. The usefulness of *Johns Hopkins Evidence-Based Practice for Nurses and Healthcare Professionals: Model and Guidelines*, Fourth Edition, is underscored by its simplicity and its language, which is free of research jargon. Students may use the book as a required textbook along with a foundational nursing research text. As each topic is discussed, readings are selected to supplement the topic.

Research at the baccalaureate level is often offered as a 3-credit course. The purpose of this course is to introduce students to the scientific process with emphasis on its application in nursing. The steps of the research process may be presented along with major research designs, including experimental and quasi-experimental studies, surveys, and descriptive and qualitative designs. The course emphasizes developing an understanding of the logical process of research, carrying out studies of nursing interest with the necessary scientific rigor, and critically reading and incorporating research into practice.

For example, students may complete assigned readings on threats to internal validity and an assigned research article. They can then spend class time discussing the threats and an overview of all threats provided as a summary of the class content. The application of content to research articles engages students. Students can use the same article discussed with the threats to highlight information recorded on the JHEBP research appraisal tool.

Students in some programs use the JHEBP tools during class as interactive exercises. For example, during the discussion of the purpose of research, students apply the section on developing an answerable EBP question using the PICO format (Patient, Intervention, Comparison, Outcomes) on pages 88–90 of the book to identify a clinical concern. Students may use the JHEBP research and nonresearch appraisal tools when critiquing studies for in-class exercises and for homework assignments.

Conducting an individual or group EBP project as a final learning activity for an undergraduate research course may develop skills for students to use after graduation in clinical practice. One way to involve nursing students with an actual clinical issue is to have them work with registered nurses from affiliated healthcare organizations to generate practice questions of concern. Faculty often find organizations' EBP committee chairs helpful in establishing this collaboration. Figure 2.1 includes EBP topics identified by affiliating hospitals. Students participate in an EBP project on a patient care unit and may cite their contribution in their portfolio. An overview of an EBP project that could be added to the course syllabus is included in Figure 2.2 with the grading rubric (Figure 2.3). Students often report that the actual EBP project is fun, and they appreciate application of these principles to practice.

Figure 2.1   EBP Questions From Affiliating Healthcare Organizations

- What is the best practice for utilizing computerized information systems to improve hand-off communication involving high-risk medications when transferring patients?
- What is the most reliable and valid sedation assessment tool for pediatric ICU patients?
- What is the patient's/family's perception of healthcare workers' professional image/dress?
- What is the smallest size peripheral IV catheter that can be used in an adult for blood transfusion and prevention of hemolysis to the cells?
- What interventions have been implemented to manage disruptive behavior between and among professionals in the workplace?
- What are the best strategies to decrease errors in pathology specimen labeling?
- Does double-check verification of medication prior to administration decrease medication errors?
- What are the best chest pain stratification tools/guidelines for use at triage?
- What is the best practice for a feeding model that supports the infant's neurological development and is easily translatable to staff and parents?
- What is the best practice to improve International Venous Thromboembolism (I-VTE-1) compliance?
- What are the safe interventions in preventing falls in the ambulatory setting compared to current practice?
- How long can an asymptomatic peripheral intravenous access remain in place prior to site rotation among adult inpatients?

Figure 2.2   Guidelines for Group Evidence-Based Practice Project

Purpose:

The purpose of the EBP project is to have the student demonstrate skills in applying research to practice. This is a group exercise. The PICO and all tools are available on the course website.

Procedures:

Students will work in teams of three to six. Each group will:

  a. Identify a topic of interest using the PICO form. Topics may be clinical, management, or educational nursing practices.

  b. Conduct a literature search on the chosen topic and select appropriate articles for critique. Include at least eight articles of evidence. Critique each article using the JHEBP tools. Include copies of the articles in the final report.

  c. Complete an individual summary tool that includes limitations, level, and quality of evidence.

  d. Complete a synthesis and recommendations tool that includes practice recommendations.

  e. Evaluate each member's contribution to the group project, including your own.

The evidence report should be organized in a narrative report in the following way:

  1. Abstract

  2. Introduction (overview of clinical problem area)

  3. Purpose

     • Relevance to nursing

     • Significance of project

  4. Methodology

     • Description of literature review

     • Types and level of evidence found

     • Volume of research in the area

  5. Brief results

  6. Conclusion and implications for nursing (practice recommendation)

  7. Reference list in APA format

  8. Appendices:

     • Individual Evidence Summary Tool

     • Synthesis and Recommendations Tool

     • Copy of each piece of evidence reviewed, with appraisal forms for each article

     • Peer reviews in individual, sealed envelopes

Figure 2.3 Grading Rubric for Baccalaureate-Level EBP Project	
	Possible Points
Executive summary	8
Introduction	
Methodology	
Brief description of results	
Conclusions	
Implications	
Individual evidence table	8
Evidence is categorized correctly	
Results displayed are accurate	
Limitations are listed	
Level and strength of evidence are accurate	
Evidence summary table	9
Evidence is accurately summarized	
Practice recommendations are thorough	
Conclusions are based on the evidence presented	
Oral presentation	3
APA format is accurately used, and appendices are complete	2
(points could be deducted)	
TOTAL POINTS	30

The American Association of Colleges of Nursing's *Essentials of Master's Education in Nursing* states that master's education must prepare the graduate to translate evidence into practice (www. aacnnursing.org/Portals/42/Publications/MastersEssentials11.pdf). In addition, accrediting agencies such as The Joint Commission and Magnet Recognition Program® have incorporated research and evidence-based practice (EBP) as necessary components of nursing practice for organizations to ensure healthcare excellence.

Similar to undergraduate programs in nursing, the master's program should weave the EBP paradigm throughout the curriculum rather than include it only in one or two courses. Whereas undergraduates focus on beginning scholarship for practice, master's students are prepared to use new knowledge and begin to translate it into practice. They use the same process as undergraduate students, but the expected outcomes of the course requirements are at a higher level. Whereas undergraduate-level students may be expected to develop an EBP question and critique an individual article related to that topic, at the master's level, students may be required to assess the state of the science on a topic related to their practice specialty. The varied backgrounds and abilities of incoming students present a challenge in graduate education. Some students matriculate with a recent research course and thorough understanding of the basics of EBP. Others need to be reminded of, or taught for the first time, the basic content of EBP. All graduate research courses should focus on the translation of research to practice settings.

Application of Research to Practice Course

One example of a master's-level course is "Application of Research to Practice." This required core research course prepares students to translate the best available evidence into practice as they serve in advanced-level roles in healthcare organizations. The course includes a review of the research process (including theoretical framework, design, analysis, and research design hierarchy), research critique, rating and synthesizing the strength of evidence, decision-making for practice, research and research translation opportunities (outcomes, evaluation research, quality improvement, cost-effectiveness analysis), risk adjustment, measurement, research ethics, and organizational change. Although some of this material would have been covered at the undergraduate level, the emphasis in the master's course is on applying the concepts to evaluating and translating evidence related to advanced practice.

The course outcomes for the "Application of Research to Practice" for the master's nursing student are:

1. Apply knowledge from the sciences to the advanced practice of nursing through utilization of an EBP model to answer a clinical, administrative, or educational nursing question.

2. Demonstrate advanced knowledge of the research process and research designs through critique of research and nonresearch evidence.

3. Differentiate among designs for nursing research in terms of principles, variables, validity, sampling, procedures, strengths and limitations, and identification of gaps in knowledge.

4. Analyze the various approaches to the measurement of variables and collection of data.

5. Discuss the statistical methods used to analyze research data.

6. Use the research process to address problems within areas of advanced clinical nursing practice and nursing systems by synthesizing the state of knowledge on a specific topic and recommending strategies to test interventions for improvement.

Among many course requirements, two learning activities focus specifically on EBP skills and knowledge. The first is a group research critique, which requires students to demonstrate the ability to critically evaluate a scientific paper based on their knowledge of the research process and information on elements of a critique that they learned in the class. For this assignment, students are divided into two groups. Each group reads two assigned articles prior to the class session. One article is considered primary, and the second is considered secondary. Group 1 presents its designated primary article for discussion, answering questions from Group 2, which has also read the article and will share (secondary) information related to the article. Then Group 2 presents its designated primary article for discussion, fielding questions from Group 1, which, again, has read the article and will share its secondary response. The questions will vary based on the selected article, but examples of primary and secondary questions are presented here.

Questions for Primary Article:

1. What is the study purpose?

2. For this study, define "cases" and "controls."

3. Is the study prospective or retrospective?

4. What statistical analyses were applied to the study data?

5. What are the clinical implications of the study findings?

Questions for Secondary Article:

1. Was the literature review comprehensive?

2. What were the study variables? Were they clearly defined?

3. How were the independent and dependent variables measured?

4. Were the measurement instruments reliable and valid?

5. Can the results be generalized?

The second key assignment for the course is the state of the science paper. This paper is designed to reflect the student's ability to evaluate and synthesize current and relevant data providing the state of evidence on a specific nursing issue. The assignment requires the student to conduct a thorough literature search, critically appraise the current evidence on the identified nursing issue, summarize that evidence, and develop a plan to implement evidence-based recommendations from the evidence review (Figure 3.1). In addition to the paper, students are required to submit a JHEBP Individual Evidence Summary Tool (pages 316–318 in the book) and Synthesis and Recommendations Tool (pages 320–323 in the book). Students submit the paper in two parts so that they are able to receive feedback on their definition of the clinical problem and their search strategy. They review the literature and make recommendations in the second part of the paper. Students are encouraged to choose topics for the research state of the science paper that are in their specialty area.

Integration of EBP Into Master's Clinical Courses

Identifying, using, and evaluating evidence related to practice, including standards of care (guidelines and protocols), is a focus of master's degree clinical courses. Students search various sources of evidence for current practice guidelines and are encouraged to download them to their electronic device. During the weekly clinical conferences, students present and discuss relevant findings, including evaluation of use in their practice environments.

Use and evaluation of evidence in the clinical practicum is not confined to the direct-care clinical courses. For example, health systems management students may review and evaluate the evidence used in the recommendations from the National Academy of Medicine reports or position statements written by professional organizations, such as the American Nurses Association or the American Organization for Nursing Leadership.

Master's-Level Scholarly Project

In addition to the core research course, graduate students may be required to write an article to submit for publication or develop a poster for display. The purpose of the assignment is to investigate a complex clinical problem. Students are expected to synthesize and integrate knowledge gained from current and previous master's-level coursework and apply that knowledge to a clinical problem by utilizing the best available scientific evidence. Projects may be developed over the course of three academic semesters. In the first semester, the students may develop a PICO statement on a topic or problem of interest. In the second semester, the students may review the literature on this topic. In the final semester, the students may develop and present a poster on their project. The poster reflects and builds upon the students' clinical question and PICO statement developed in the first semester. It also builds upon the evidence-based review of the second semester's literature, evaluating the literature's strength and implications.

Figure 3.1   State of the Science Paper Guidelines and Grading Rubric

Part I (five-page limit, including abstract, excluding references): 10 points total

Title (one page) and abstract (one page, double-spaced) **(1 pt)**

- Title: The title reflects the variables and population.
- Abstract: The abstract includes information about the problem, background, and purpose of the paper.

Introduction **(8 pts)**

- The problem and rationale are clear.
- The purpose of the paper is explicitly stated.
- The introduction presents a case for the need to study the topic and its relationship to nursing.
- All major concepts are introduced and defined.
- The search strategy, keywords, inclusion criteria, and number and types of evidence reviewed are included and adequately described.

Organization/Formatting **(1 pt)**

- There is a logical flow of ideas and proper grammar and spelling.
- The paper, including citations and reference page(s), uses APA format correctly throughout.

Part II (10-page limit, excluding abstract, references, and appendixes): 90 points total

1. An abstract—with a conclusion related to the state of the science—has been added. **(5 pts)**

    2. The state of the science on the nursing issue is described with sources of evidence critically reviewed and synthesized. The evidence is summarized in the JHEBP Individual Evidence Summary Tool (found on pages 316–318 in the book). **(10 pts)**

    3. The strengths and limitations of the current evidence are described. The evidence base for practice change is clearly supported, or the identified gap in evidence is compelling and significant. **(25 pts)**

    4. Implications for nursing research/practice/policy are identified and linked to the level of evidence from the preceding synthesis of literature. **(25 pts)**

    5. Recommendations for translating evidence to practice or initiation of further research are identified and linked to the level of evidence from the preceding synthesis of literature. This should include a feasible plan for implementation of EBP, an identification of key stakeholders and an appropriate interdisciplinary team to assemble, and a brief plan for outcome analysis, including independent and dependent variables and a method of statistical analysis. **(25 pts)**

Part 4
Doctoral Education

Doctoral education in nursing today follows two distinct degree paths: Doctor of Philosophy (PhD) and Doctor of Nursing Practice (DNP). Both build nursing knowledge and develop specialized skills, and both focus specifically on the discipline of nursing. More importantly, at the level of doctoral study, students are challenged to critically evaluate the complete body of science and evidence available to answer important nursing-related questions and solve nursing practice problems. Students are pressed to analyze and synthesize information from many disciplines and sciences in addition to nursing. The body of evidence to be considered is large and broad; as a result, doctoral students can benefit from conducting their search and evaluation using a framework such as the one presented in *Johns Hopkins Evidence-Based Practice for Nurses and Healthcare Professionals: Model and Guidelines*, Fourth Edition. The JHEBP approach helps doctoral students analyze and synthesize evidence by providing a structure and process to organize, evaluate, track, and present the evidence in a logical, integrative way.

PhD education focuses on research, which is the discovery of new knowledge. Students ask questions about nursing, its practice, and its problems for which no answers are available or complete. The work is characterized by clean design, control of extraneous variables, careful execution, reliable and valid measurement, and precise evaluation.

DNP education focuses on application of new knowledge in practice. The students ask questions about nursing practice and problems. This work is characterized by careful design but differs from the work of the PhD students in several significant ways. The DNP students are engaged in solving practice problems by applying or translating the discoveries of researchers, ensuring fidelity of this translation of evidence, and closely monitoring the outcomes of translation. For the DNP, confounding variables are everywhere, and evaluation is commonly conducted using data collected for other purposes (www.aacnnursing.org/Portals/42/Publications/DNPEssentials.pdf).

A Primer on EBP

The JHEBP Model can serve as prereading on the topic and process of evidence-based practice (EBP). For doctoral students who lack prior knowledge and experience with EBP, the JHEBP Model is an appropriate place to begin. For students whose education proceeds directly from entry to practice to a career in research, the text can provide exposure to the types of problems and concerns facing the practicing nurse.

The appendix in this guide includes a sample DNP scholarly project curriculum outline that is aligned with the current American Association of Colleges of Nursing's *Essentials: Core Competencies for Professional Nursing Education* Advanced-Level Nursing Education Sub-competencies (AACN, 2021). The frameworks used to design this curriculum outline are the *JHEBP Model PET Pathway* (Dang et al., 2021) and *Implementing the EBP Competencies in Academic Settings: EBP Integration in Graduate Programs* by Melnyk & Fineout-Overholt (2019). The curriculum outline utilizes all the JHEBP Model's tools to help doctoral students progress through the process in a systematic manner. Additional tools are highlighted in the following sections with examples of how they have been utilized in practice.

Using the PICO in Education

The PICO tool is helpful for staff engaged in the work of EBP. Introduced early in the EBP process, the PICO tool guides the work of a team approaching problem-solving. The same tool that staff find useful to focus efforts has also been found to hamper the process of inquiry for doctoral students. A premature focus on a solution leads to a search of the evidence constructed to validate the proposed intervention, rather than discovering the most effective one based on rigorous evaluation of evidence. Such consensual validation delays and confounds true understanding of the options for solving important clinical problems.

Searching, Reviewing, and Appraising the Literature

Once students identify the problem or question, identifying the evidence for review and appraisal is critical to the investigation of the problem and must be approached systematically. Figure 4.1 is an example of a grading rubric that could be used for the search strategy assignment.

Several of the tools are helpful in introducing doctoral students to the complexity of appraising evidence and reviewing the literature. PhD students create original scholarship in the writing of the dissertation's review of the literature. This is the foundation for the question posed, the variables measured, and the hypotheses tested. The complexity of this work challenges critical thinking and organization. The JHEBP Model supports both by providing process and structure. DNP students describe a clinical problem including its background and significance, conduct an appraisal of the evidence, and propose a strategy to improve outcomes. This work is predicated on a comprehensive, methodical evaluation of the evidence that can be supported using the model.

Organizing and Presenting the Evidence

The Individual Evidence Summary Tool, found on pages 316–318 in the book, can be helpful as a template to organize the large and complex body of information relevant to the research question or practice problem. Because of the tremendous variability in the nature and the quality of evidence available to drive practice improvement (opinion statements, institutional guidelines, case studies, and research), the model is particularly useful for DNP students. The Synthesis and Recommendations Tool, found on pages 320–323 in the book, can aid doctoral students in managing the rating of individual studies and items of evidence. This tool allows students to combine all pieces of evidence from each level and synthesize that material.

Doctoral students, like practicing nurses, need to be able to discriminate levels of quality and rigor across disparate documents and to present the findings reported in this context. The students need to create a logical argument for the strategy proposed to address the clinical problem. Synthesis of evidence based on an assessment of quality, consistency, and applicability is key for the students to make an overall recommendation and the critical decision about which evidence should be translated to solve the practice problem in a particular setting.

The individual evidence summary helps manage this complex assignment. A sample is provided in Figure 4.2.

Teaching Models and Metrics

Evaluation of EBP models can also be useful as a strategy to deepen understanding of the translation process and critical thinking. Students can compare and contrast similarities and differences in model development, terminology, and application. They are easily engaged in discussions about how various models have been used and under what circumstances, both in a theoretical and a practical sense. The JHEBP Model has a distinct third phase labeled *translation* that is not explicit in other EBP models. This third phase establishes a direct connection to the work of the DNP, which is translation.

One example of an assignment for the DNP program is found in Figure 4.3. This assignment is at the end of the DNP students' first semester and is the culmination of the EBP course. The assignment requires that students choose an EBP model and use it as the basis for development of a manuscript or paper on a topic that includes the clinical problem statement, problem significance, clinical practice question, search strategies, grading of evidence, synthesis of evidence, and proposal for translation.

Figure 4.1   Evaluation of Search Strategy—100 Points (or could be any percentage of 100)

1. Succinctly describe the issue or problem. 10 points

2. What are your search terms? List them in order and in any combinations used. Did you use any controlled vocabulary, such as subheadings or MeSH terms? 20 points

3. Where did you go for your evidence? Name and describe the databases and other resources. Describe any hand-searching or footnote searches. Give rationale for your choices. 20 points

4. What type of output did you receive from your search? Too much or too little? How did you refine your search? Did you add terms, use Boolean operators, limit to certain study designs? 20 points

5. What inclusion and exclusion criteria did you use to keep or discard a piece of evidence? 20 points

6. Document your final search—dates, terms (all of the strategy above, from 2–5). How did you arrive at an acceptable output of evidence? 10 points

Figure 4.2   Organizing and Presenting the Evidence Using the Individual Evidence Summary

First Author	Year	Level of Research (or non-research) Evidence	Sample Composition & Size	Results/ Recommendations	Limitations	Rating Strength/ Quality
Stoll	2010	Non-experimental (retrospective, observational)	9,575 infants < 28 weeks gestational age (GA) and VLBW (< 1500g) Birth date January 1 2003–December 31 2007 at NICHD Network Centers	Rates of survival to discharge increased with increased GA. Infants at lowest GAs were at greatest risk for morbidities. Most early deaths occur at 22 and 23 weeks GA (85% and 43% respectively). Majority of infants with GAs > = 24 weeks survive but with high rates of morbidity	All infants born at NICHD centers, possibly negatively skewing survival rates and positively skewing morbidity rates	III/A
Anderson	2004	Non-experimental (cross-sectional survey)	142 US NICUs Infants < 1500g	Wide range of SpO2 guidelines. "Gradient of risk" toward less retinal ablation surgery with SpO2 < 98% in first two weeks of life ($p < 0.05$). Statistically significant lower rate of >/= stage 3 ROP with SpO2 </= 92% after first two weeks of life. Randomized controlled trial needed to determine O2 administration, O2 saturations, and development of ROP for the very preterm infant	No sample size given. No upper limit of SpO2 identified to reduce risk of ROP in very preterm infants. Variety of pulse oximeters used. Alarm settings not surveyed	III/B

| Figure 4.2 | Organizing and Presenting the Evidence Using the Individual Evidence Summary | | | | | |

First Author	Year	Level of Research (or non-research) Evidence	Sample Composition & Size	Results/ Recommendations	Limitations	Rating Strength/ Quality
Birenbaum	2009	Quasi-experimental	Single-center; infants less than 1500g Two groups: 1) birth year 2002 ($N = 73$) 2) birth year* 2005 ($N = 73$) * After quality improvement process initiated	Significant reduction in incidence of chronic lung disease in 2002 birth year group compared to 2005 group: 46.5% in 2002 vs 20.5% in 2005	Quality improvement process instituted in 2005 was multi-factorial (avoidance of intubation, adoption of new lower target pulse oximeter limits, and early use of nasal continuous positive airway pressure therapy)	II/A
Chow	2003	Quasi-experimental	Single-center; infants less than 1500g $N = 421$ Data collected over five-year period (1997–2001)	Differences in clinical practices after implementation of O2 policy affected the rates of retinopathy of prematurity (ROP): 12.5% to 2.5% in 1997 and 2001 respectively Similar reduction in ROP laser therapy for same time period	Many potential confounders Insufficient evidence to support cause and effect relationship between educational process, change in clinical practice regarding SpO2 target guidelines, and decreased ROP rates	II/A
Deulofeut	2007	Quasi-experimental	All inborn infants < 1250g born from January 2000 to December 2004 ($N = 497$) Two groups: 1) Born 1/00 to 12/02 (target SpO2 92–100%) ($N = 297$; 140 male) 2) Born 1/03 to 12/04 (target SpO2 85–93%) ($N = 200$; 101 male)	Practice change 1/03: target SpO2 85–93% Analysis by gender: rate of ROP, CLD, and length of stay better for female infants than males in period 2 compared to period 1 Neither gender had increased neurological morbidity or short-term detrimental effects with lower SpO2 targets	Potential basis for different effect size seen with gender in very preterm infants not described	II/A

Figure 4.2		Organizing and Presenting the Evidence Using the Individual Evidence Summary				
First Author	Year	Level of Research (or non-research) Evidence	Sample Composition & Size	Results/ Recommendations	Limitations	Rating Strength/ Quality
Deulofeut	2006	Quasi-experimental	502 infants </= 1250g admitted to single center NICUs (two) during period 1/00–12/04: 1) 300 infants born 1/00 to 12/02 (target SpO2 92–100%) 2) 202 infants born 1/03–12/04 (target SpO2 85–93%)	Rates of ROP, supplemental oxygen at 36 wks post-conceptual age (PCA), and use of steroids for CLD significantly lower in group 2 Higher Mental Developmental Index scores and Psychomotor Developmental Index scores in group 2 No differences between groups in rate of NEC, IVH, or PVL	Partial data available on actual periods of time at various O2 saturation levels Educational program and intention to treat led to a different approach to oxygen therapy and increased awareness of healthcare personnel	II/A
Askie	2003	Multicenter, double-blind, randomized, controlled trial	358 infants < 30 weeks GA who remained dependent on supplemental oxygen at 32 weeks PCA Two groups: 1) standard saturation (91–94%) 2) high saturation (95–98%)	Primary outcomes: growth and neuro-developmental measures at 12 months corrected age (PCA) No significant differences in growth or frequency of major developmental abnormalities Targeting a higher O2 saturation range in extremely premature infants dependent on supplemental oxygen conferred no significant benefit with respect to growth and development Higher target O2 saturation ranges results in increased burden on health services (40% increase in # infants still receiving O2 therapy at 36 weeks PCA and a 78% increase in # infants receiving supplemental O2 therapy after discharge)		I/A

Figure 4.2		Organizing and Presenting the Evidence Using the Individual Evidence Summary				
First Author	Year	Level of Research (or non-research) Evidence	Sample Composition & Size	Results/ Recommendations	Limitations	Rating Strength/ Quality
Payne	2006	Quasi-experimental	16 centers 12-225 VLBW admissions in 2001 2001 rate of BPD (baseline) compared to 2003 rate (outcome year) after implementation of potentially best practices (PBP) to reduce incidence of BPD	13 PBP to reduce BPD identified based on published evidence and expert opinion No change in BPD rate 2001 vs 2003 among centers Successful initial implementation of PBP did not guarantee continued implementation Multi-institutional collaboration facilitated development and implementation of PBP to reduce BPD	Multifactorial difficulty recruiting support for PBP among centers Non-uniform implementation of specific PBP by participating centers ("institution-specific" PBP choice)	II/B
Sears	2009	Quasi-experimental	Consecutive infants born 8/1/05–7/31/07 (N = 190) and admitted to a single Level III intensive care nursery Two groups by birth year: 1) 8/1/05–7/31/06 (standard O2 sat target 95–100%) 2) 8/1/06–7/31/07 (new O2 sat target 85–92% for infants < 34 wks GA, 92–97% for infants >/= 34 wks GA)	Incidence of ROP 35% in group 1, 13% in group 2 Stage 3 ROP disease decreased from 11% to 2% Threshold disease (just prior to ablation need) decreased from 7% to 1% Statistically significant differences also seen in mode of O2 delivery, sepsis, and O2 at discharge Small change in oxygen effectively reverses deleterious effect of hyperoxia on developing retina Further randomized, prospective clinical trials needed to evaluate zone and stage of ROP because they provide important information for extremely premature infants	No separation of results for very preterm babies (less than 28 wks GA)	II/A

Figure 4.2   Organizing and Presenting the Evidence Using the Individual Evidence Summary

First Author	Year	Level of Research (or non-research) Evidence	Sample Composition & Size	Results/ Recommendations	Limitations	Rating Strength/ Quality
STOP-ROP Multicenter Study Group	2000	Randomized, controlled trial	649 infants with pre-threshold ROP in one eye and median pulse oximetry saturation < 94% in room air Randomized to two groups: 1) Conventional (N = 325); pulse oximetry target 89–95% 2) Supplemental (N = 324); pulse oximetry target 96–99% Each group continued in arm for at least two weeks or until study eye reached ophthalmic endpoint	Supplemental O2 at pulse oximetry saturation readings of 96–99% did not decrease progression of pre-threshold ROP and did not improve growth or eventual retinal outcome at 50 weeks Supplemental O2 increased risk of adverse pulmonary sequelae including pneumonia, worsening chronic lung disease, need for O2, diuretics, and continued hospitalization at three months PCA No difference in growth and developmental milestones between groups Modest deleterious effect of supplemental O2 on CLD in infants with more severe lung disease at baseline	Predictive value of various definitions of pre-threshold ROP have not been systematically studied Unclear explanation for observation that those babies excluded from the trial due to pulse ox saturations > 94% in room air had a strong tendency toward better outcomes than those infants in the high-saturation study group (protective effect of high spontaneous saturations) No data to suggest that higher O2 sat levels are safe for the immature eye that does not have ROP	I/A
Tin	2001	Non-experimental (retrospective, observational)	295 infants < 28 weeks GA surviving infancy (Northern England) Two groups based on target O2 saturations in first eight weeks of life: 1) 88–98% 2) 70–90%	Infants who received supplemental oxygen to maintain O2 saturation of 88–98% for first eight wks of life developed severe ROP requiring cryotherapy four times as often as babies only given enough O2 to maintain O2 saturations of 70–90% No difference in survival of infancy or development of cerebral palsy; similar neurodevelopmental outcome at one year No association between much lower target O2 saturations and adverse effects on growth between birth and discharge O2 policy differences had impact on amount of ventilator support provided and therefore the total cost of care before discharge	Need RCT to establish if other unrecognized confounding factor was responsible for results	III/A

| Figure 4.2 | Organizing and Presenting the Evidence Using the Individual Evidence Summary ||||||

First Author	Year	Level of Research (or non-research) Evidence	Sample Composition & Size	Results/ Recommendations	Limitations	Rating Strength/ Quality
Vander-Veen	2006	Quasi-experimental	323 infants </= 1250g and/or < 28 wks GA Two groups: 1) Birth 6/1/00–5/31/03 2) Birth 6/1/03–5/31/04* * new oxygen saturation policy (alarm limits lowered to 85–93%)	Rate and severity of ROP in the year after the oximetry alarm policy change to the rates in the immediately preceding three years: Rate of pre-threshold ROP in infants during year after O2 alarm policy change compared to the three years prior to the change: 5.6% vs 17.5% (68% reduction in pre-threshold ROP) Simple change in oximeter alarm parameters in the first few weeks of life may decrease the incidence of pre-threshold ROP and lower rates of unfavorable visual outcomes caused by ROP	No long-term data on benefits and potential risks of lowering oxygen saturation targets, especially on neuro-developmental outcomes	II/A
Wright	2006	Quasi-experimental	Three NICUs Inborn infants 500–1500g 191 infants before implementation of PROP, 159 infants after implementation of PROP	Significant reduction in rate of threshold disease after implementation of PROP = physiologic reduced oxygen protocol (O2 saturation levels by pulse oximeter 83–93%) No change in brain or lung damage, or infant mortality with lower arterial oxygen saturation protocols	Sample size too small to draw conclusions Inclusion criteria = BW < 1500g (low risk of developing ROP) Modest changes in oxygen saturation target for treatment group compared to control group No conclusion about importance of reducing fluctuations in arterial oxygen saturation vs lowering of saturation limits No baseline characteristics of the infants	II/B

Figure 4.2   Organizing and Presenting the Evidence Using the Individual Evidence Summary

First Author	Year	Level of Research (or non-research) Evidence	Sample Composition & Size	Results/ Recommendations	Limitations	Rating Strength/ Quality
Hintz	2011	Non-experimental (retrospective, observational)	411 infants < 25 weeks EGA born 1999– 2001 (epoch 1) 405 infants born < 25 weeks EGA born 2002– 2004 (epoch 2) All data prospectively collected from the NICHD NRN Generic Database and follow-up study Comparison of survival, perinatal characteristics, neonatal interventions, and morbidities between two epochs	Adverse neurodevelopmental outcomes at 18–22 months' corrected age Early childhood outcomes for infants born at < 25 weeks EGA were unchanged between the two periods	Did not include a normal birth weight control group Not a population-based cohort	III/A

Figure 4.3   Guidelines for Evidence-Based Practice Paper

Students will write a final paper on EBP regarding the clinical problem identified and the practice initiative(s) selected. This paper will be evaluated (see criteria below) and represents 50% of the final course grade.

Criteria for Evaluation

1. The prevalence and severity of a health problem is defined.   **5 points**

2. Evidence related to this problem and related practice initiative(s) is evaluated, graded, and synthesized. Search details are provided. The evidence strengths, limitations, and gaps in knowledge are identified.   **30 points**

3. A theoretical framework that describes the relationships among the concepts related to the selected clinical problem or evidence is presented.   **15 points**

4. The need for future research regarding the health problem and practice initiative(s) is clearly described. (There is a clear link between the problem and the evidence, and there is a clear need for a practice initiative/change.)   **10 points**

5. An EBP framework is defined.   **10 points**

6. A plan is presented to translate the evidence into practice using the identified EBP framework as a guide.   **10 points**

7. Strengths and limitations of the translation plan are discussed.   **10 points**

8. A research summary table and reference list in APA format follow the main body of the paper.   **10 points**

Part 5
Professional Development for Healthcare Organizations

Instilling the Basics

One of the primary goals of evidence-based practice (EBP) education within a healthcare organization is to identify a variety of teaching strategies that will enable healthcare professionals at any level to develop the necessary skills to create or evaluate clinical interventions and make everyday practice decisions.

Because educational planning across an organization is a major undertaking, forming a small group or steering committee that can oversee this process is highly recommended. Committee members should include individuals who are familiar with research, EBP, staff education, and management within the organization. Representation from a variety of backgrounds and disciplines can be beneficial not only to identify the appropriate teaching methods and content, but also to identify and obtain the necessary resources (staffing, finances, equipment) that will ensure the program's success. Frequent attendance by steering committee members at key leadership meetings within the organization is an essential strategy for informing administration and gaining needed support for EBP education.

Building EBP Capacity

Building EBP capacity refers to ensuring that staff have the necessary knowledge, skills, and resources to conduct EBP projects and to translate best practices into the clinical setting. Educational opportunities and experience gained through participation in interprofessional EBP teams are often the most effective strategies for developing EBP competencies. EBP mentors can also provide additional support and a safe space for learning new EBP skills.

Learning Needs Assessment

The first step in developing an EBP educational plan is to perform a learning needs assessment specific to the healthcare organization. There are several ways to do this. One of the easiest ways to perform a needs assessment is through a staff survey. Ask survey participants to rate their level of proficiency in performing a literature search, obtaining evidence, and evaluating research articles. There are several validated tools in the EBP literature that can facilitate this process. Also, query them about their previous participation in quality improvement projects, EBP projects, and other initiatives designed to improve patient outcomes. Using an online survey platform can make it easier for participants to respond and for surveyors to collate the data.

Focus groups are a second approach. Bring together small groups of staff to obtain feedback on what they need to be successful in conducting EBP projects. In this forum, the leader can provide the group with an overview of the EBP process, discuss the needed skills, and obtain feedback from participants. A third approach to performing the needs assessment is to discuss staff learning needs with clinical specialists, educators, and unit-based instructors. These individuals work closely with bedside clinicians and can be a valuable resource in identifying the learning needs of staff. They can also provide valuable information about which educational strategies will work best for their respective departments or clinical areas.

No matter which approach or combination of approaches is used, taking the time to identify learning needs upfront allows the design of an EBP educational program that meets the specific needs of staff. For example, if staff members have identified the need for improved computer and literature search skills, build more time into the educational plan to develop these skills. In addition, gather staff feedback on learning needs after each educational activity to redirect teaching efforts, ensuring that the educational plan is meeting participants' needs.

Identification of Teaching Methods

Various EBP teaching methods can be used within the healthcare setting. This section discusses four approaches: 1) small-group mentored approach, 2) workshop approach, 3) online learning, and 4) developmental approach. Regardless of the teaching method employed, the following content is always necessary:

1. Definition and importance of using EBP (Chapter 1)

2. The EBP process and how each step is used (Chapter 3)

3. The method for developing an EBP question (Chapter 4)

4. Different types of evidence and how to locate each (Chapter 5)

5. Ways to appraise research and nonresearch evidence (Chapters 6 and 7) using the EBP research and nonresearch evaluation tools

6. Technique for translating EBP findings into practice (Chapter 8)

Small-Group Mentored Approach

The small-group mentored approach has been found to be effective in teaching EBP because it allows participants to become familiar with the EBP process and tools while simultaneously completing a real-life project. In this approach, a small group of staff, usually from the same area of practice, is brought together to explore a practice question of importance to the group's clinical setting. When participants select the practice question themselves, they are often more motivated to use the EBP process to obtain the answer. One of the mentor's first responsibilities is to help the group refine and narrow the EBP question, using the EBP Question Development Tool, so it can be efficiently searched.

Once the EBP question is developed, the group is then mentored through the EBP process by one or two mentors who are experienced in EBP. The EBP Work Plan can track the group's progress. Regular group meeting times are established for one to two hours each. Mentors provide the didactic content (listed in the preceding section) in the first one or two sessions.

Mentors then help participants gather and analyze the evidence. To gather the evidence, mentors can search the literature and provide articles for the group. Or several group members, depending on their experience level, can perform the search and gather articles. Other group members can gather additional evidence, such as initiating contact with other healthcare organizations to determine the community standard related to the EBP question, checking with professional organizations for policy statements or position papers, or contacting experts on the topic. The mentor should also advise the group on strategies to track the literature search and screening processes.

Appraising evidence is often best accomplished using a group approach. The group approach generates discussion, brings multiple perspectives to the table, and sparks the critical thinking process. Two simple approaches to using groups can be employed. First, you can involve all group members to read and appraise each article or piece of evidence. Second, you can divide the work of reading and appraising the articles among the group. If the second approach is used, divide the articles in such a way that at least two members of the group read each article. Mentors need to read all the articles to lead the group through the appraisal process. In addition, mentors need to ensure that group members understand how to use the EBP research and nonresearch appraisal tools to determine the strength and quality of the evidence under review. It can be helpful to have the whole group read an article and appraise as a team to discuss the process and organically identify questions or areas for clarification. After individual group members read the EBP articles, they present them to the entire group. Using the Individual Evidence Summary Tool (pp. 316–318), the group discusses each article, determines the strength and quality of the evidence, and identifies key results/recommendations. Mentors can complete this tool during the discussion by using a laptop connected to a projector so that all group members can track the key points. Once the individual articles are appraised, the group then completes the Synthesis and Recommendations Tool (pp. 320–323) and determines the overall strength and quality of the body of evidence. The laptop and projector approach can also be used for this form. Based on the strength and quality of evidence, the mentor helps the group decide whether a practice change is warranted. If a modification should be made, the mentor helps the group translate the change into practice, such as by protocol change, guideline, or teaching tool.

Workshop Approach

EBP workshops are an excellent way to train a large number of staff and to develop EBP mentors. One of the most effective ways to help participants gain experience with EBP is to design the workshop so that it simulates an actual EBP project. We have the most success with the one-day workshop format. Chapter 2 provides the sample one-day workshop format. Didactic content is taught during the first part of the workshop, followed by an interactive computer and group-evidence appraisal in the afternoon. The class participants then determine whether a practice change is warranted based on the available evidence.

The workshop approach, however, adds a degree of complexity to identifying an EBP question that is important to the entire class. One strategy for identifying a question is to poll the participants prior to the workshop to identify a common question or theme that can be used, such as pain management, falls, or pressure ulcer prevention. Another strategy is to identify a common problem across the organization (perhaps alarm management or medication administration) that can be used as an EBP question. Once the question is identified, workshop organizers can then search the literature for articles to be appraised as part of the evidence-appraisal portion of the workshop.

Participants are given at least two articles to read before the workshop so that they can complete the evidence review. Articles are divided among participants so that at least two read the same article. During the workshop, participants learn to use the Research Evidence Appraisal Tool and the Nonresearch Evidence Appraisal Tool, and they discuss the articles and other evidence in a group that is led by workshop organizers. Participants evaluate findings, and the group makes a preliminary determination about whether a change in practice is needed.

The learning needs assessment may indicate that class participants need time to enhance computer skills to support the EBP process. How this portion of the workshop is conducted depends on the resources available to the healthcare organization. Having computer time available allows students to conduct a hands-on literature search related to the practice question. Library specialists may be enlisted to teach this section. If logistics make this difficult, this section may be taught by lecture and discussion format.

Longer and more intensive approaches, two- to five-day workshops may be offered for mentors and EBP champions. These individuals often need more in-depth exposure and time to master the content and interact with the EBP leadership team. You can find a sample agenda for a two-day workshop in Figure 5.1.

A fast-track EBP educational approach that includes six two-hour sessions designed to fit easily into a work schedule may also be effective for a single unit or department. The sessions can be conveniently offered over the lunch hour or during another time the unit identifies. The sessions are offered in shorter blocks of time and should be conducted over a limited period for best results, such as one session per week for six weeks. This also allows participants time between sessions to review content and read articles. The sample agenda for the fast-track sessions is found in Figure 5.2.

Online Learning

Some healthcare facilities require flexibility in staff education. An online asynchronous course may be effective for those organizations. The Johns Hopkins Nursing Center for Evidence-Based Practice offers an online course that walks the learner through the EBP process. Upon completion of the course, the participant will be able to:

1. Address clinical, educational, financial, and administrative problems using the JHEBP Model.

2. Identify an EBP problem and formulate a PICO question.

3. Participate in EBP projects.

4. Lead EBP projects.

5. Search and appraise the literature.

6. Generate best evidence recommendations and translate these to the practice setting.

7. Implement change using the JHEBP Model.

For more information about the online course or to register to take the course, see https://www.ijhn-education.org/node/.

Developmental Approach

The developmental approach to teaching EBP skills involves conducting projects through the departmental committee structure of the organization. This approach promotes the involvement of clinical staff because membership on committees such as Standards of Care and Quality Improvement are often composed of frontline clinicians.

Developing an EBP project in the committee and using a portion of committee time to learn and implement the various steps of the PET process can energize committee members because it allows dedicated time for them to focus on a topic of interest. As part of the meeting, the committee can discuss relevant practice issues and use the EBP Question Development Tool to identify and refine an EBP question. Conducting several EBP projects throughout the year, as part of the committee's routine objectives, is an excellent way to teach bedside EBP skills and improve practice. Initial projects can be conducted by committee members themselves. *Johns Hopkins Evidence-Based Practice for Nurses and Healthcare Professionals: Model and Guidelines,* Fourth Edition, can serve as a step-by-step guide in developing the committee's EBP project. As committee members gain more experience in the process, other bedside clinicians can be invited to join future EBP projects to learn the process.

An agenda item devoted to EBP support allows participants to benefit from the collective expertise of the committee while designing and conducting EBP projects in their own departments or units. The committee can also serve as a clearinghouse for communication of EBP projects throughout the organization. Keys to success include dedicating time during the committee meeting to provide updates on EBP projects in progress (see EBP Work Plan in Figure 11.1 in the book); developing a standardized method for narrative reporting of EBP projects; providing a template for poster presentations; and developing a web page to post information related to EBP projects, including contact information, so interested individuals can learn more about the projects.

To disseminate EBP education throughout an organization, it is essential to develop EBP mentors. These mentors can participate by providing workshops, leading project teams within their departments, and encouraging others to develop EBP questions or projects. Providing EBP education to central (organization-level) committee members—such as the central Standards of Care, Education, and Research committees—is a good place to start. Membership on central committees is usually composed of staff members who hold leadership positions in departments. Providing EBP education to committee members enables these individuals to take the information back to their departments, lead departmental EBP project teams, and mentor others. Requiring each central committee to participate in EBP projects throughout the year also helps build the EBP skills of central committee members and gives them experience in leading or participating in EBP project groups.

Another approach to developing EBP mentors is the EBP fellowship program. See Figure 5.3 for EBP fellowship objectives.

Fanning the Flame

The work of healthcare occurs primarily in the service setting, where traditional coursework is seldom a feasible option. Strategies that incorporate EBP into the fabric of existing processes and structures are most successful in promoting and sustaining a culture of EBP.

Chapter 2 can guide nurse leaders and top administrators as they learn how to create a supportive EBP environment. The chapter provides examples for development of mission statements, managing change and transitions, and overcoming barriers to fostering an EBP culture. These can be used as examples in small-group work sessions that enable learners to develop supportive strategies, as relevant to their organizations.

Educators using this book to instruct healthcare leaders on methods to promote and sustain EBP can demonstrate the use of teachable moments to provide mentorship in developing EBP skills and competencies. Examples that can be used in discussion group format include journal clubs, preceptor as EBP mentor, incorporation of EBP content into core continuing-education offerings, training-reinforcement activities, committee support for EBP projects, and facilitated protocol development and review.

Journal Clubs

Journal clubs, which are wonderful tools to enhance lifelong learning, have great utility for building organizational capacity for EBP. Journal clubs develop skills and build confidence in searching for evidence and using evidence-based information resources, critically appraising both research and nonresearch evidence, synthesizing evidence, and making recommendations for practical application of findings. Through reading and sharing of ideas, participants work collaboratively to assess a piece of evidence that has direct relevance to their practice. EBP journal club leaders can build on the learning objectives in Chapters 4 through 8 to help club members develop essential EBP skills and competencies. Club members can use tools provided in the appendices to structure development of a question of mutual interest, evidence appraisal, and summarization of evidence.

Key factors for success include leaders who release club members from patient-care responsibilities during designated meeting times, a club leader well-versed in EBP techniques to provide consistent mentorship, and administrative support to procure and distribute evidence. Leaders may also want to explore the use of technology, including online discussion boards and video conferencing recordings, to facilitate an offsite or asynchronous experience that may allow for greater participation.

Preceptor as EBP Mentor

The bedside, or point of care, provides the perfect venue for capturing teachable moments. Supporting new nursing staff during the first year is often the responsibility of a preceptor or other nurse who has a defined role in unit-based orientation and education of new staff. Preceptor training in EBP principles and concepts can enhance informal, incidental, interpersonal, and interactive learning during the orientation process and throughout the first year of practice. The power of the "how we do things here" mentality is strong. Clinical experiences and interpersonal interactions of the preceptor-learner dyad provide a convenient forum for infusing EBP at the earliest stages of workforce development. The preceptor has the valuable opportunity as a clinical role model to assist the newly hired nurse to think critically, to pose important clinical questions, and to base patient care decisions on evidence. Preceptors with strong EBP skills make it clear that EBP is part of the nursing culture. Key factors for success include training preceptors to model expected EBP behaviors and skills and taking advantage of each teaching encounter to impart the importance of seeking out and translating evidence to patient care.

Core EBP Continuing Education

There are various ways to incorporate EBP into the continuing education activities of the organization. As with initial learning experiences, different formats can be used, depending upon unit scheduling requirements. Flexibility is the key, and learners who have developed basic EBP skills should be encouraged to participate in the development of advanced workshops.

Self-learning activities range in complexity from printed self-learning packets to narrated PowerPoint slides to online courses developed by an instructional designer. These self-guided learning activities can be used for orientation, as an adjunct for other training, or for yearly refreshers.

Monthly lunch-and-learn sessions are also becoming increasingly popular to reinforce continuing education because they do not require nurse leaders to release staff from patient care responsibilities. Scheduled during staggered lunch periods, these sessions can reinforce content over time and provide targeted learning-application activities to be completed between sessions.

Facilitated Protocol Development

Most organizations have a defined process for protocol or policy development, review, and revision. These activities present first-rate opportunities to build organizational capacity for EBP by cultivating EBP skills and competencies in the teams that actually develop, review, and revise clinical practice standards. *Johns Hopkins Evidence-Based Practice for Nurses and Healthcare Professionals: Model and Guidelines,* Fourth Edition, can take teams step by step through the EBP process to guide protocol development. Keys for success include making sure that clinical questions are important to the content of the protocol; assigning an EBP mentor or fellow as a consistent resource to the protocol development and review team; and communicating the results of the EBP review, along with education surrounding new or revised protocols.

Conclusion

Infusing EBP knowledge and skills throughout a healthcare organization involves a comprehensive educational plan that employs multiple educational strategies, based on the needs of staff and organizational resources. The key to the plan's effectiveness rests not only with the education provided and the teaching approaches used, but also with the organization's ability to build capacity through development and support of mentors both at central and departmental levels. Mentors are instrumental in helping the organization build a culture of continual learning that encourages staff to question clinical practice and promotes EBP to examine practice issues. Using a steering committee to develop and frequently evaluate the comprehensive plan can also help ensure that adequate resources are devoted to EBP training and that necessary alterations are made to the education plan to ensure its effectiveness over time.

Figure 5.1   Sample Two-Day Workshop Agenda

Day 1	Topic
8:00 a.m.–8:15 a.m.	Opening Remarks—Overview of Day
8:15 a.m.–9 a.m.	Intro to Evidence-Based Practice (EBP)
9:00 a.m.–9:45 a.m.	Johns Hopkins EBP Model and Process
9:45 a.m.–10:00 a.m.	Break
10:00 a.m.–11:30 a.m.	Appraising the Evidence
11:30 a.m.–12:30 p.m.	Lunch
12:30 p.m.–1:45 p.m.	Computer/Library Lab (distribute article packets)
1:45 p.m.–2:00 p.m.	Break
2:00 p.m.–2:30 p.m.	Computer/Library Lab—Searching Your Own Problem
2:30 p.m.–2:45 p.m.	Q and A and Review of Assignment and Format for Day 2

Day 1 ends early to allow time for participants to read their assigned articles.

Day 2	Topic
8:00 a.m.–8:15 a.m.	Opening Remarks—Overview of Day
8:15 a.m.–9:15 a.m.	How to Run an Effective EBP Meeting/Moving an Agenda
9:15 a.m.–10:15 a.m.	Mock Evidence Appraisal Group Meeting
10:15 a.m.–10:30 a.m.	Break
10:30 a.m.–11:30 a.m.	Summary and Synthesis Skill Building
11:30 a.m.–12:30 p.m.	Lunch
12:30 p.m.–2:00 p.m.	Should Practice Change Based on Evidence?
2:00 p.m.–2:15 p.m.	Break
2:15 p.m.–3:15 p.m.	Creating a Supportive EBP Environment
3:15 p.m.–3:45 p.m.	Program Wrap-up and Evaluation (Day 2)

Figure 5.2   Fast-Track EBP Educational Sessions

Topic and Time Suggestion	Objectives
Session #1 (30 minutes)	
Introduction to EBP	Define EBP and describe the importance of EBP
Session #2 (30 minutes)	
EBP Model	Discuss the Johns Hopkins EBP Model and Guidelines (PET process)
Session #3 (20 minutes)	
Searching the Evidence	Identify and describe different types of evidence and how to locate them
Session #4 (20 minutes)	
EBP Process	Discuss the PET process in detail
Session #5 (20 minutes)	
Evidence Appraisal Tools	Describe how to use the EBP tools
Session #6 (45 minutes)	
Appraising the Evidence	Describe how to evaluate different types of evidence
Session #7 (30 minutes)	
Evaluation and Next Steps	Review expectations for the project, including getting started and translating evidence into practice

Figure 5.3   EBP Fellowship Objectives and Expectations: A Johns Hopkins Example

The EBP fellowship is designed to develop advanced EBP skills and to lead EBP initiatives at a unit, department, and hospital-wide level. The EBP fellow conducts literature reviews for selected topics, appraises existing evidence using the JHEBP Model, and convenes and manages a multidisciplinary EBP team. During the nine-month EBP fellowship (October–June), the selected individual will work two days/week on the following:

1. Lead and mentor a team (selected by the Standards of Care Committee) on an EBP project using the JHEBP Model:

    • Identify a practice issue.

    • Recruit and lead a multidisciplinary team.

    • Conduct a comprehensive literature review using search databases.

    • Complete a summary of recommendations derived from the project that considers the feasibility of evidence translation and change.

    • Draft a dissemination plan, including measurable outcomes.

    • Present results of projects at the unit, functional unit, and hospital levels.

2. With support of mentor, assess needs of department in meeting EBP.

3. Consult with Standards of Care members, as requested:

    • Assist with selection or refinement of PICO question.

    • Assist with literature search techniques.

    • Assist with education on how to appraise articles.

    • Assist with summarizing data, translating it, and disseminating the findings.

    • Consult on PowerPoint or poster display of findings.

4. Coordinate the EBP article review workshop:

    • Select a general topic, which may be clinical, administrative, or educational.

    • Search for applicable articles related to the selected topic and appraise articles prior to workshop to ensure an array of various levels of evidence, such as Levels I–V.

    • Email and assign participants to read articles prior to the workshop.

    • Confirm group facilitators for EBP workshop.

    • Conduct an evaluation of the EBP workshop and summarize evaluation results for dissemination to the EBP Steering Committee and presenters.

5. Consult with Johns Hopkins University School of Nursing (JHUSON) research classes:

    • Follow up with JHUSON students on practice questions that students are searching.

    • Attend research students' presentations and acquire EBP information for dissemination to Nursing Standards of Care members.

6. Consult with clinical leadership on other EBP topics that present throughout the year.

7. Participate in EBP educational activities, such as (but not limited to):

    • Review EBP models and development of a comparison table; be able to distinguish the JHEBP Model from other EBP models.

    • Review a module on statistics.

- Complete the online EBP modules.
- Meet with a librarian to discuss search strategies.
- Participate in EBP online module updates, panel discussions, and publishing opportunities as requested.

8. Provide 1:1 or group presentation on EBP model as requested.

9. Adhere to EBP office maintenance:

- Review and update the EBP website monthly.
- Maintain EBP information in an EBP directory.
- Maintain and update the JHEBP annotated bibliography.

Appendix

Sample DNP Scholarly Project Curriculum Outline: Evidence-Based Practice (EBP) Practice Question-Evidence-Translation (PET) Pathway and Competencies for DNP Scholarly Projects

Aligned with the current American Association of Colleges of Nursing's (AACN) *Essentials: Core Competencies for Professional Nursing Education* Advanced-Level Nursing Education Sub-competencies (AACN, 2021)

Framework: The JHEBP Model PET Pathway (Dang et al., 2021) and Implementing the EBP Competencies in Academic Settings: EBP Integration in Graduate Programs by Melnyk & Fineout-Overholt (2019)

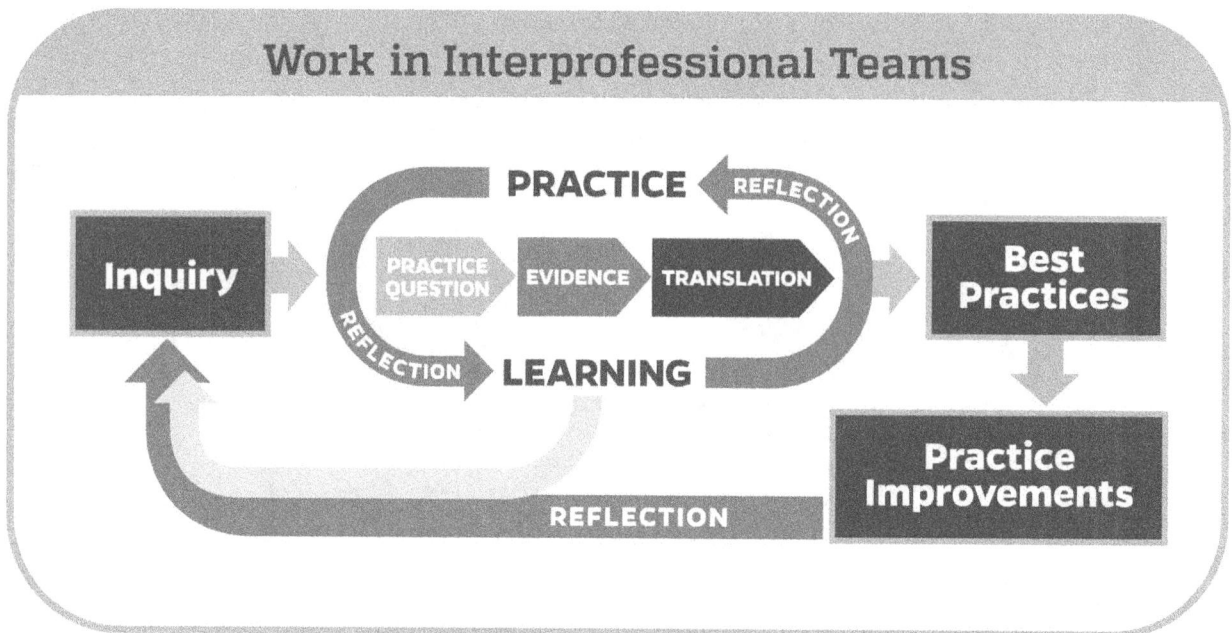

FIGURE A1 Work in interprofessional teams: The JHEBP Model for Nurses and HCPs (2021)

DNP Scholarly Project Curriculum Outline

Note: Sample plan of study for four to five 1-credit project courses including 218 practicum hours

Project Course #1: Practice Question/Problem Statement and Stakeholder Identification

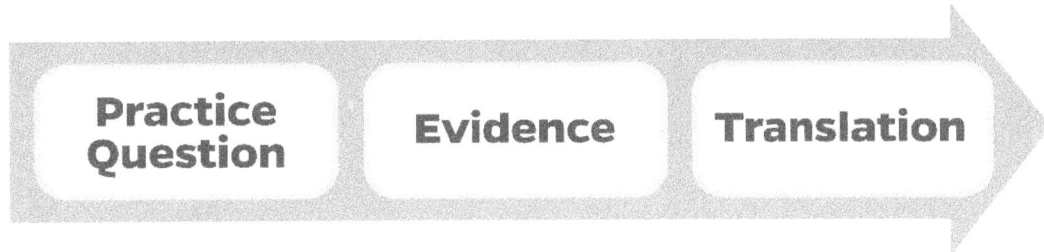

RN Competencies and Pre-requisites: Learners build upon baseline knowledge and professional practice application of the:

- AACN Essentials Entry-level (Level 1) Professional Nursing Education Sub-competencies (AACN, 2021)
- EBP Competencies #1–13 derived from pre-licensure RN program (Melnyk & Fineout-Overholt, 2019, p. 319)

Course Objectives:

- AACN Essentials Level 2 Professional Nursing Education Sub-competencies and Domains (AACN, 2021, pp. 17–58)
- Melnyk & Fineout-Overholt EBP Competencies in Graduate Programs: #14–16

Course Activities/Assignments:

- Practicum hours: 0–25 hours
- PET Pathway: Learners identify project topic/focus/problem at a specific project site and for a specific population
- Learners complete these worksheets to aid in focusing and narrowing their project approach:
  - Appendix A (see Appendix A, "PET Process Guide," in *Johns Hopkins Evidence-Based Practice for Nurses and Healthcare Professionals*, Fourth Edition)
  - Fishbone (see Figure A2 for an example; also oriented with concept map)
  - Appendix B (see Appendix B, "Question Development Tool")
  - Learners to identify their project team members/stakeholders (see Appendix C, "Stakeholder Analysis and Communication Tool")
  - Hospital/unit stakeholders, community partners, primary care practices providers, health departments/clinics, legislative policy, non-governmental organizations/non-profit organizations, etc.

- Formulate problem statement/purpose of the project focus and choice:
  - Considerations: Does this look to be human subjects research, quality improvement, and/or a process improvement?
  - Exploratory PET Pathway process: Will this be an individual or a team/group project?

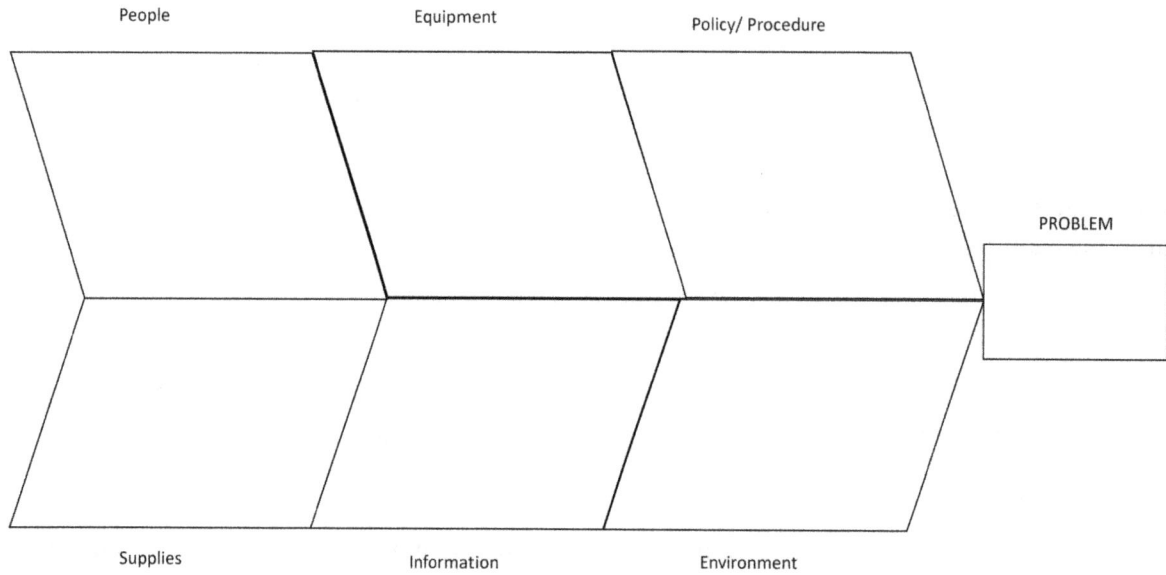

FIGURE A2 Fishbone template.

Project Course #2: Exploring the Evidence

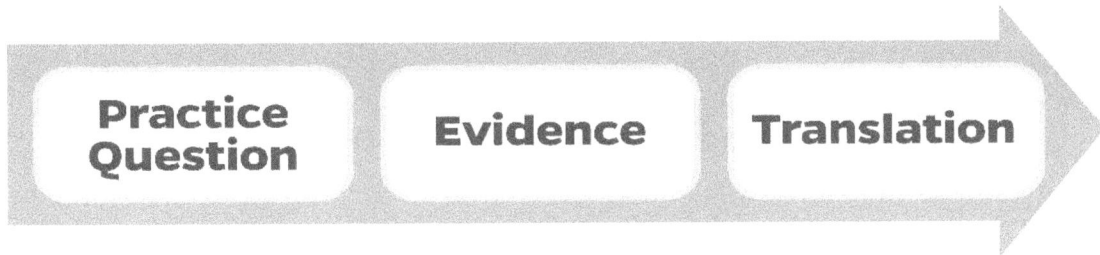

Practice Question → **Evidence** → **Translation**

- Learners explore various EBP translational models (KTA, Iowa, etc.) or use the organization's translational EBP model for the project

- Learners query and engage with the project site and stakeholders for micro data evidence supporting the need for an EBP PET project to improve patient care outcomes at that site and for the specified population, and compare this to known mesa and macro evidence

- Learners identify clinical experts/leaders specific to the project topic

- Practicum hours: 0–25 hours

- Learners explore the literature for evidence of current and up-to-date best practices and EBP methodologies, recommendations, and/or guidelines related to the project problem or topic focus

- Learners complete these worksheet tools:

  - Appendix E and F (see Appendix E, "Research Evidence Appraisal Tool," and Appendix F, "Nonresearch Evidence Appraisal Tool," for systematic searches [group work])

  - Collaborating course: Integrative Review course (see Appendix G, "Individual Evidence Summary Tool")

- Learners can now formulate (see Appendix H, "Synthesis and Recommendations Tool")

- Continuation of achieving Melnyk & Fineout-Overholt EBP Competencies in Graduate Programs: #14–16

Project Course #3: Connecting the Evidence for Project Translation

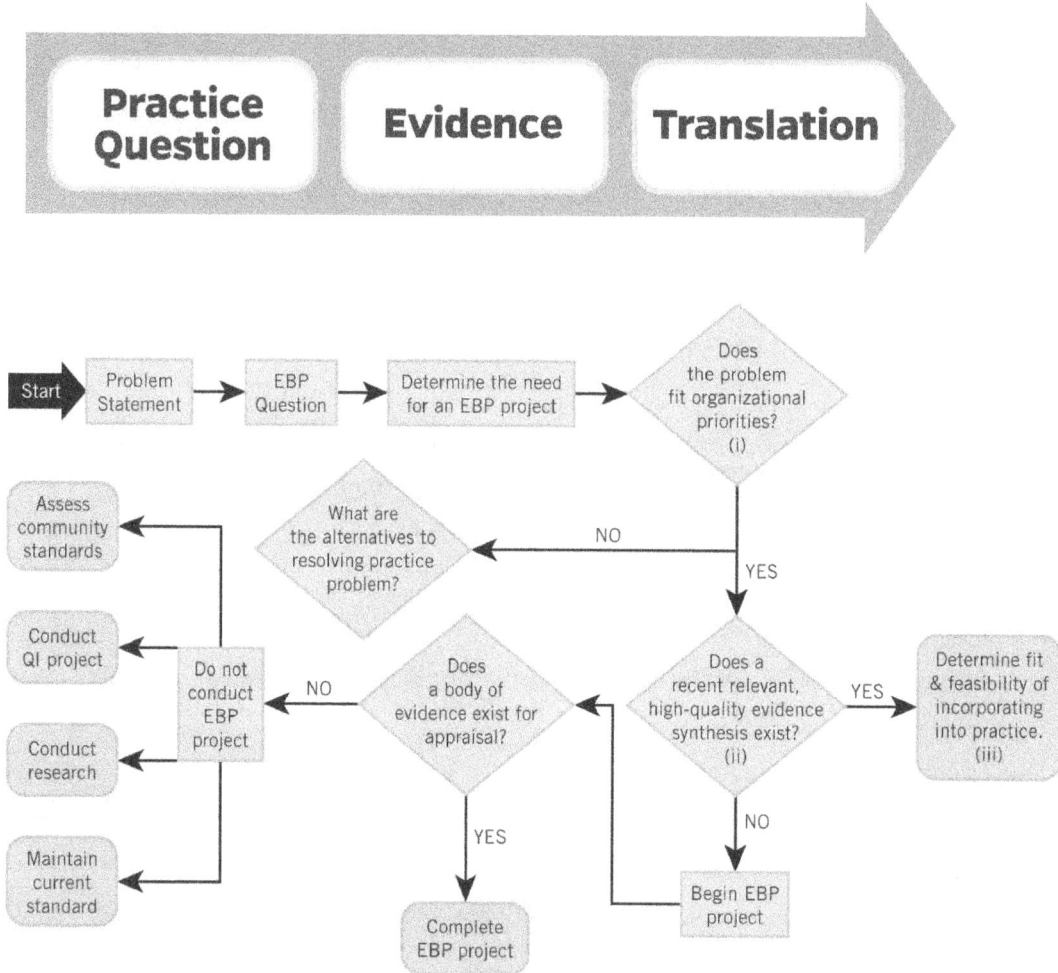

Key to the EBP Project Decision Tree:

i. Organizational priorities include unit, department, hospital, and programmatic.

ii. Team critically evaluates an existing evidence synthesis to ensure not only quality, but also that the findings are applicable to their setting and population and have been completed recently enough to represent the current environment. Make practice changes based only on high to moderate strength of syntheses of evidence, rather than on a single, low-quality evidence synthesis.

iii. Refer to the JHEBP Model and Guidelines for Nursing and Healthcare or the online EBP modules for assistance in determining fit, feasibility, and appropriateness.

FIGURE A3   Decision tree to determine the need for an EBP project represents DNP process.

Course Objectives:

- AACN Essentials Level 2 Professional Nursing Education Sub-competencies and Domains (AACN, 2021, pp. 17–58)
- Melnyk & Fineout-Overholt EBP Competencies in Graduate Programs: #14–16, 17–19, and 23

Course Activities/Assignments:

- Learners engage with project site stakeholders, leaders, and clinical experts specific to the project topic, population, and preliminary EBP intervention (QI) or proposal
- Practicum hours: 56 hours
- Learners will: Critically appraise, synthesize the literature, and integrate the findings to develop an EBP project action plan for a healthcare intervention or a process improvement ("translating evidence to construct a strategy or method to address a problem and designing a plan for implementation and actual implementation when possible," AACN, 2021, p. 24)
- Learners will formulate project SMART goals or aims reflecting the problem statement, PICO question, and/or purpose statement for the project action plan and consider the impact of patient care/provider practice on either a direct QI/(live) or indirect project (exploratory/PI)
- Learners develop a work breakdown structure plan and/or a Gantt chart to reflect the project timeline and identify the strengths, weakness, opportunities, and threats of the project and risk-mitigation strategies
- Learner will identify the data collection and methodology plan to evaluate data outcomes measurements (QI or PI), such as the tools or surveys or aggregate data/rates collection to present the results, assess feasibility and sustainability, and/or expert critique and review for future QI
- Learners utilize and continue to refine:
  - Appendix A: Continue to work on
  - Appendix I (see Appendix I, "Translation and Action Planning Tool")
  - Appendix C (see Appendix C, "Stakeholder Analysis and Communication Tool")
  - Formulate an A-3 Tool (see Figure A4)
- Learners will present the developed action plan to the appropriate approval unit (agency or university IRB, etc.) for review to translate the project's action plan

JOHNS HOPKINS
MEDICINE

A3: Patient Satisfaction

A3 Project Leader_____
Rev. Date_____

Define
Background:

Objective / Goal:	Team Members:

Key Metrics:

Measure (Pre-Post Measures as annotated graph)
Insert graph of performance

Analyze: Identifying & Prioritizing root causes of failures and "bright spots"

Improve: High-level timeline with action steps taken

Control: Achieving High Reliability

FIGURE A4 A blank A-3 template.

Project Course #4: Translation of Project Action Plan

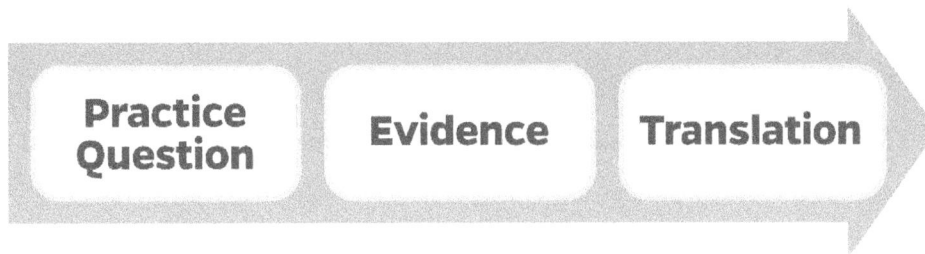

Course Objectives:

- AACN Essentials Level 2 Professional Nursing Education Sub-competencies and Domains (AACN, 2021, pp. 17–58)
- Melnyk & Fineout-Overholt EBP Competencies in Graduate Programs: #14–16, 17–19, and 23

Course Activities/Assignments:

- Learners engage with project site stakeholders, leaders, and clinical experts specific to the project topic, population, and preliminary EBP intervention (QI or Proposal) for active project translation
- Practicum hours: 56 hours
- Appendix A: continue work on
- Learners will launch/implement the developed action plan (Aims) and begin data collection methods; translation leaders will translate either the direct or indirect project action plan and evaluate the impact of patient care/provider practice

    1. QI/Traditional DNP Project: Live implementation of Aims Interventions

        - Data methods/gathering align with QI: pre/post intervention design or aggregate data collection (chart review or tool usage, etc.)

    2. Exploratory Project/PI:

        - Implementation of action plan of project aims and measure project outcomes (QI)
        - Query experts on feasibility and sustainability (PI)
        - Learners can develop and distribute a virtual module/bundle of a proposal: various resources
        - AHRQ bundle sets, proposed tools/flowcharts, educational in-service modules, assistance with grant proposal/submission/NGOs, legislative activity, etc.
        - Bundle for Magnet® qualifications or continual certification

- Translate the data analysis and methods: Appraise and assess pre/post tools, surveys, and/or critiques from expert clinicians/team members on the developed action plan (the material, bundle, tool, grant application, policy, etc.)

- Begin to assess and critically integrate post critique feedback and analyze "what changes are needed for improvement" (see Figure A5) and revise accordingly

Model for Improvement

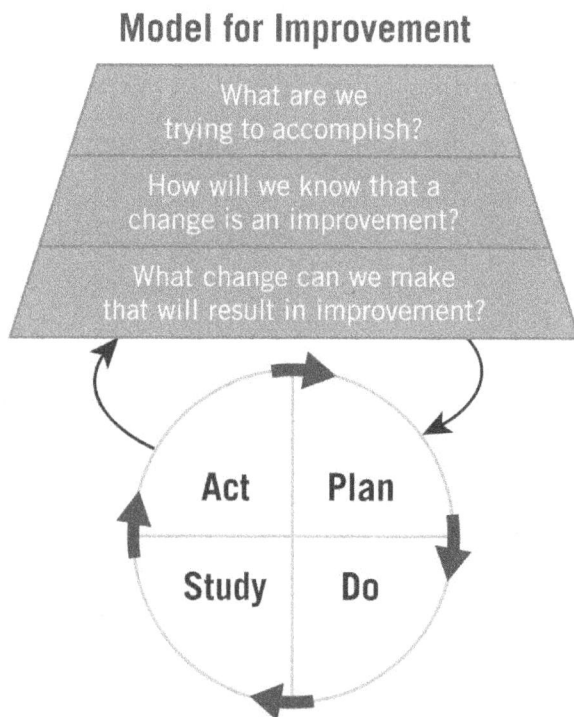

FIGURE A5   Model for improvement.

Project Course #5: Evaluation of the Translation and Dissemination

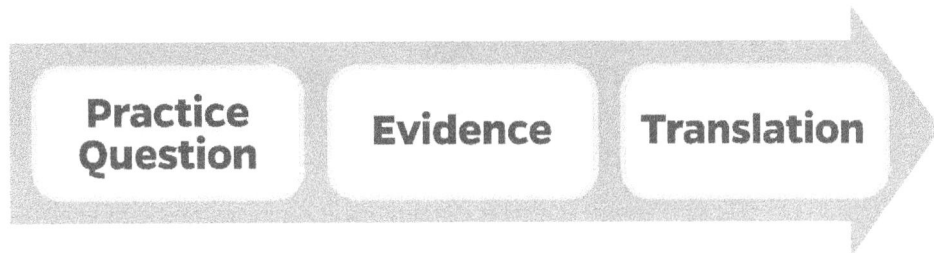

Course Objectives:

- AACN Essentials Level 2 Professional Nursing Education Sub-competencies and Domains (AACN, 2021, pp. 17–58)
- Melnyk & Fineout-Overholt EBP Competencies in Graduate Programs: #14–16, 17–19, and 23, 20, 21, & 24; demonstrate competencies in all 24 EBP Integration Competencies

Course Activities/Assignments: In collaboration with 808 Data Analyses course

- Learners engage with project site stakeholders, leaders, and clinical experts specific to the project topic, population, and preliminary EBP intervention (QI) or proposal for evaluation and dissemination
- Practicum hours: 56 hours
- Learners will conduct an "evaluation of the outcomes, process, and/or experience" of the action plan experience/work (AACN, 2021, p. 24)
- Translation evaluation: Learners will discover and evaluate either the direct or indirect project action plan and analyze the impact of patient care/provider practice
- Appendix A: continue work on
- Examine and evaluate the evidence of the data through analysis and evaluation methods. Appraise and assess pre/post tools, surveys, and/or critiques from expert clinicians/team members on the developed action plan (the material, bundle, tool, grant application, policy, etc.): The measures used that aligned with the action project's aims or goals and align with the project's purpose/problem statement and/or PICO question
- Systematically assess and critically integrate post critique feedback and analyze "what changes are needed for improvement" (refer to Figure A5) and revise accordingly
- Dissemination and presentation to stakeholders:
  1. Poster and/or PowerPoint presentation to stakeholders and/or agency leaders

2. Explore, describe, and disseminate the project's results and outcomes on patient care outcomes: Will the project become the site's best practices or is there continued revision needed? (PDSA cycle)

   a. If QI: Will the EBP best practice intervention become standard practice and/or be incorporated into the project site's patient care or provider practice/education? (feasibility and sustainability)

   b. If a PI: Further query, revisions, and/or actions needed to secure a future QI project?

- Learners: final paper or manuscript as per appropriate journal (student can choose)

- Appendix J (see Appendix J, "Publication Guide")

Reference Materials

American Association of Colleges of Nursing. (2021). *The essentials: Core competencies for professional nursing education,* rev. February 21, 2021. Author.

Dang, D., Dearholt, S. L., Bissett, K., Ascenzi, J., & Whalen, M. (2021). *Johns Hopkins evidence-based practice for nurses and healthcare professionals: Model & guidelines* (4th ed.). Sigma Theta Tau International.

Melynk, B., & Fineout-Overholt, E. (2019). *Evidence-based practice in nursing & healthcare* (4th ed.). Lippincott Williams & Wilkins, Wolters Kluwer Health.

www.ingramcontent.com/pod-product-compliance
Lightning Source LLC
Chambersburg PA
CBHW061821210326

41599CB00034B/7077